Understanding breast reconstruction

GW00503970

This booklet is for you if breast reconstruction after surgery is being considered for you. It has been prepared and checked by cancer doctors, other relevant specialists, nurses and patients. Together they represent an agreed view on this cancer, its diagnosis and management, and the key aspects of living with it.

If you are a patient, your doctor or nurse may wish to go through the booklet with you and mark sections that are particularly important for you. You can make a note below of the main contacts and information that you may need quickly.

Specialist nurse/contact names | Family doctor ....

.... | ....

Hospital | Surgery address

.... | ....

.... | ....

.... | ....

Phone .... | Phone ....

Treatments .... | Review dates.................

.... | ....

.... | ....

If you like, you can also add:

Your name ....

Address ....

Understanding breast reconstruction – key points in this booklet

This booklet tells you about breast reconstruction, and the benefits and problems you might experience with this kind of surgery. These two pages sum up the main points, and show which pages to turn to for more information.

What is breast reconstruction? Page 7

An operation to restore the shape of the breast after a mastectomy or lumpectomy operation.

When can breast reconstruction be carried out? Page 8

It can be carried out either at the same time as breast cancer surgery or later. If you have had radiotherapy it is necessary to wait some months to allow the skin in the treatment area to recover.

How is it carried out? Page 9

There are two main types of breast reconstruction:

- using an implant

- using a 'tissue flap', in which muscle and skin from your back or abdomen is transplanted to the chest to form the reconstructed breast.

What materials are used? Page 13

Breast implants are basically textured silicone shells, and can be filled with saline (salt water), silicone gel, or triglycerides (a substance similar to body fat).

Silicone implants – are they safe? Page 14

Experts advised the Department of Health in 1996 that there is no good reason to stop using silicone implants, and this advice is still followed. But it is important to talk through any concerns you have with your breast care nurse or surgeon before having an implant.

Breast reconstruction using muscle and skin flaps
Page 15

This procedure is used where a lot of skin and muscle has been removed from the breast, or where tissue expansion for an implant is not suitable.

What can you expect from breast reconstruction?
Page 24

Every effort is made to get the best result, and a reconstruction should give you a balanced appearance when wearing a bra. But it is impossible to achieve a perfect match with the remaining breast. The photos on page 00-00 give some idea of what can be achieved with different types of breast reconstruction.

Recovery after breast reconstruction, and possible complications Pages 26-27

These pages list some practical things that can be done to ease recovery and avoid or reduce the complications that can arise.

Finding a surgeon Page 30

It is essential to find a reputable and experienced surgeon to carry out your breast reconstruction. This section includes some questions you might want to ask.

For more information

The back of this booklet lists answers to common questions (page 33), BACUP's services (page 35), other useful organisations (page 36), some recommended reading (page 39), and a fill-in form for questions to ask your doctor, breast care nurse or surgeon (facing inside back cover).

3 Bath Place, Rivington Street, London, EC2A 3JR

BACUP was founded by Dr Vicky Clement-Jones, following her own experiences with ovarian cancer, and offers information, counselling and support to people with cancer, their families and friends.

We produce publications on the main types of cancer, treatments, and ways of living with cancer. We also produce a magazine, *BACUP News,* three times a year.

Our success depends on feedback from users of the service. We thank everyone, particularly patients and their families, whose advice has made this booklet possible.

Administration 0171 696 9003
Cancer Information Service 0171 613 2121 (8 lines)
Freeline (outside London) 0800 18 11 99
Cancer Counselling Service 0171 696 9000 (London)
BACUP Scotland Cancer Counselling Service
0141 553 1553 (Glasgow)

British Association of Cancer United Patients and their families and friends. A company limited by guarantee. Registered in England and Wales company number 2803321. Charity registration number 1019719. Registered office 3 Bath Place, Rivington Street, London, EC2A 3JR

Medical consultant: Dr Maurice Slevin, MD, FRCP
Editor: Peter Chambers
Cover design: Alison Hooper Associates
Acknowledgements
Sylvia Denton, OBE, MSc, RGN, RHV, ONCCert, FRCN senior clinical nurse specialist in breast care at the Royal Hospitals NHS Trust, for the original draft of this publication
Robert Carpenter, BDS, MS, FRCS,
Mrs Dalia V. Nield, FRCS (Ed)
Royal Marsden NHS Trust, for permission to use their 1994 booklet on breast reconstruction as a source of information for this booklet
Royal Marsden NHS Trust Breast Unit, for advice on the information included
Breast Cancer Care
Mr Nigel Sacks, MS/FRCS FRACS
Mr Ian Fentiman, MD, FRCS
Mr A G Nash, FRCS
Dr Susan Mayor, for additional research and editorial support.

Typeset and printed in Great Britain by Lithoflow Ltd., London
ISBN 1-901276-08-2

Contents

Introduction   6

What is breast reconstruction?   7

Why consider breast reconstruction?   7

When can breast reconstruction be carried out?   8

How is breast reconstruction carried out?   9

Reconstruction using an implant   10

Materials used in breast implants   13

Silicone implants – what are they and are they safe?   14

How long do silicone implants last?   15

Breast reconstruction using muscle and skin flaps   15

Reconstructing the nipple   23

Surgery to the other breast   24

What can you expect from breast reconstruction?   24

Recovery after breast reconstruction   25

Radiotherapy after breast reconstruction   26

Possible complications after breast reconstruction   27
    Immediate problems   27
    Longer-term problems   29

Finding a surgeon   30

Checking your breasts after reconstruction   31

Mammography after reconstruction   32

Common questions   33

BACUP's services   35

Useful organisations   36

Recommended reading   39

Questions to ask your doctor, breast care nurse or surgeon (fill-in page)   *facing inside back cover*

Introduction

This booklet has been written for women who have undergone or are about to undergo a mastectomy, so may be considering breast reconstruction. It aims to help you understand more about what breast reconstruction is and the possible benefits and problems you might expect from this type of surgery. It also covers some of the physical and emotional problems having breast reconstruction may bring and makes some suggestions for helping you to cope with them.

This booklet also provides general information about different methods of reconstruction and practical matters such as immediate and long-term after-care.

In a booklet of this size it is not possible to give every detail. So it is very important that you discuss all aspects of the issue before making any decisions. Every woman's needs are different and only you – together with your doctor and any family and friends you wish to involve – can decide what might be best for you. Give yourself plenty of time to weigh up the potential benefits and disadvantages of breast reconstruction before making a decision.

> **This booklet is for women who have had or are considering breast reconstruction after mastectomy**

What is breast reconstruction?

Breast reconstruction is an operation to replace breast tissue lost during mastectomy or lumpectomy, restoring the breast shape. The aim is to match as closely as possible the remaining natural breast by creating a breast 'form' with an implant which is placed beneath the skin and muscle that covers your chest, or by using muscle from another part of your body. A combination of these techniques is used in some women.

Your doctor will advise you on the technique most suitable for you. It will depend on:

- the amount of tissue removed from your breast
- the quality of the tissue at the planned operation site
- whether or not you have had radiotherapy to your breast
- your general health and body build
- your choice and preference.

Nipple reconstruction is also possible, usually as a separate operation once the reconstructed breast has settled into its final shape.

Why consider breast reconstruction?

Not surprisingly, any woman finds it difficult to come to terms with the loss of a breast. Up to a half of all women having mastectomy choose to have breast reconstruction, either at the time or afterwards.

Benefits of reconstruction:

- in clothes (or underwear or swimming costume), your appearance will be similar to what it was before mastectomy
- even without clothes, you may feel better with a permanent breast mound restoring your natural shape

- you will not have to wear an external artificial breast (prosthesis) for the rest of your life
- it can help restore your self-confidence and feelings of femininity, attractiveness and sexuality
- it does not restrict any later treatments that might be necessary. It does not interfere with radiotherapy, chemotherapy or hormone therapy. Follow-up after the operation is no more difficult and any recurrence of cancer in the area can still be detected easily.

Limitations of reconstruction:

- it will not restore precisely the breast appearance and shape you once had
- your new breast will lack the sensitivity of your natural breast
- if you have children afterwards, you are very unlikely to be able to breast-feed with a reconstructed breast (however, it should be possible with the other breast).

It is important that you are well informed about what breast reconstruction may achieve in your case before making a decision about whether to proceed. You need to have realistic expectations about the possible result and be aware of the limitations. Most breast units have breast care nurses. If you can contact one she may be particularly helpful in providing information, based on considerable experience and understanding, about breast reconstruction in your case.

When can breast reconstruction be carried out?

Doctors differ in their views on when breast reconstruction should be performed. Some prefer to do it at the same time as breast cancer surgery while others believe it is important to wait a time, possibly a year or more after having a breast removed, before undergoing reconstructive surgery. If you have had radiotherapy you will have to wait some months before the skin in the treated area has completely recovered.

If you think you might want breast reconstruction it is a good idea to discuss the issue with your surgeon before your operation. You do not have to make a definite decision at this early stage, but if there is some chance you might want reconstruction it will help the surgeon decide on the way he or she carries out your mastectomy.

Some women find that immediate reconstruction helps them to cope with the emotions associated with the loss of a breast, and to resume normal life again.

If you are interested in having an immediate reconstruction you should discuss it with your surgeon who will tell you if it can be done. They may still recommend a delay, particularly if you are advised to have radiotherapy or chemotherapy immediately after your initial surgery.

It is also important to mention that there may be a waiting list for delayed breast reconstructive surgery because of the limited number of surgeons experienced in this field.

How is reconstruction carried out?

There are two main types of breast reconstruction:

- reconstruction using an implant of some kind
- 'tissue flap' reconstruction, in which muscle and skin from your back or abdomen is transplanted to the chest to form the reconstructed breast.

Reconstruction using an implant

1) Breast reconstruction under the skin (subcutaneous)

This type of reconstruction is possible when a woman has the breast tissue removed but the skin and nipple can be preserved. It is only suitable for women with fairly small breasts. An implant is placed beneath the skin to replace the lost breast tissue.

This kind of reconstruction is suitable for women who have certain types of breast cancer. Rarely, it is used for those who have a high risk of developing breast cancer, to try to prevent it happening (prophylactic mastectomy).

The scar which results from this type of reconstruction may be on either side of the nipple and continue sideways around it, or run in the crease under the breast.

The advantage of this type of reconstruction is that it usually looks good and is simple to carry out. However, some surgeons are concerned that problems may occur later on with this method of reconstruction – tiny deposits of cancer cells may remain or develop in the nipple and areola areas and may continue to grow.

2) Breast reconstruction under the muscle (submuscular)

This is a simple form of breast reconstruction in which an implant is placed beneath the muscles covering the chest. This method of reconstruction may be suitable if you have fairly small breasts. It is not possible if you have had a radical mastectomy (as you will have no chest muscle remaining), are large-breasted or have had radiotherapy, because your skin is unlikely to stretch enough to accommodate a big enough implant.

The scar from this type of operation is usually side-to-side or at an angle following the line of the original mastectomy scar. The advantage of this method is that it generally looks good and is a simple procedure. The disadvantage is that the implant can change shape slightly or move as the overlying muscle contracts.

Breast reconstruction using an implant

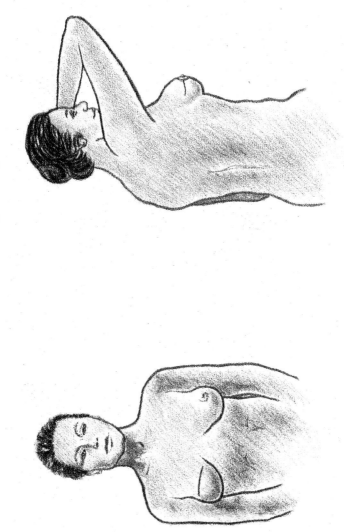

The scar may run across the breast, as shown here, or in the crease under the breast.

3) Breast reconstruction using tissue expansion

Breast reconstruction involving tissue expansion can provide very good results and avoids the need for radical surgery involved in using tissue flaps. However, it may take a much longer time to complete than other methods, and some women find this frustrating.

This method makes use of the ability of your skin to stretch. Skin is surprisingly elastic – just think how much the abdomen expands during pregnancy.

How it is done

This type of reconstruction may involve two operations. In the first, an expandable implant with a valve for filling (like an empty balloon) is inserted under the chest muscle. This is expanded over a few months by injecting a sterile salt water (saline) solution, under local anaesthetic during weekly or fortnightly visits to the out-patients clinic. You may feel a pressure sensation during this procedure but most women find it not too uncomfortable. The process will continue until the size is slightly larger than your remaining breast.

After several months the inflatable silicone bag is removed. A permanent implant is then inserted during a second operation, after expansion of the skin. The implant will match the size of your own breast and the previous over-expansion will allow it to lie on the chest wall with a more natural droop.

An alternative method of reconstruction using tissue expansion involves a silicone implant which has an inflatable inner chamber. This method avoids a second major operation. After being inflated over several weeks and left over-inflated for a further period of several weeks, it is deflated, via the valve, by extracting some of the salt water to a size to match that of your remaining natural breast. A small operation, usually carried out under local anaesthetic, is then performed to remove the valve. This usually requires only a short stay of perhaps one day in hospital.

Some discomfort may be experienced when the expander is being inflated, causing the breast to feel tight and hard. This usually lasts only a day or so after each inflation. If the discomfort is acute tell your doctor. He or she may remove some of the fluid, and inflate the implant more slowly.

This type of reconstruction is suitable and acceptable for many women. But if you have had radiotherapy your skin will probably have lost a lot of its elasticity and so tissue expansion may not be possible.

Materials used in breast implants

Breast implants are basically textured silicone shells and can be filled with saline (salt water), silicone gel or triglycerides (a substance similar to body fat). Saline has the advantage of not causing significant problems if it leaks out into the body. However, saline-filled implants do not have the natural feel of silicone-filled implants so provide a less realistic reconstructed breast.

Silicone implants are very commonly used in the UK. The silicone filling provides a natural feel to the reconstructed breast. However, there have been some concerns about possible health risks if silicone leaks from the implant. If a silicone implant ruptures, surgery is needed to remove the implant. Like saline, silicone implants obscure X-rays, making follow-up mammography slightly more difficult. It is possible to get a good mammogam of a breast containing an implant but the radiographer should be informed.

Because of some concerns about silicone-filled implants, a number of other products are being evaluated including triglyceride-filled implants.

Although silicone implants are the most commonly used in this country, there have been some concerns about them in recent years. The next two sections have been added to explain the situation.

Silicone implants – what are they and are they safe?

These implants are essentially bags of silicone gel enclosed in a thin silicone rubber case. They are designed to feel soft and flexible, like a natural breast. Silicone implants have been used for many years for breast enlargement and were very popular until reports of ruptures, leaks and infections. Some women feared they had developed autoimmune disorders, such as rheumatoid arthritis, or even cancers as a result.

Most problems have been associated with liquid silicone injections where the compound is simply injected into the breast, rather than with implants. Silicone **injections** are now banned in the US and in the UK. No link has been found between silicone **implants** and cancer in humans. The American advisory body on drugs – the Food and Drug Administration (FDA) – banned the use of silicone implants several years ago when the doubts were first raised. They are now being used again, but only for women in clinical research studies. A statement from the American National Institutes of Health current in October 1997 stated: 'There is no convincing evidence that a silicone implant induces cancer or autoimmune disease.'

In the UK, the Department of Health asked a group of medical specialists to assess the safety of silicone implants. After careful review of all available information they concluded that there is not enough scientific evidence to stop using them. A report published in 1994 said 'there is no evidence that implants increase risk of disease'. The advice is often reviewed, and a specialist group was due to report to the Department of Health in the spring of 1998.

It is important to talk through any concerns you have with your breast care nurse or surgeon before you have an implant. You could ask them to tell you if there has been any change in the official advice on the safety of silicone implants.

At the moment operations involving breast implants in the UK are recorded in a central registry so that any problems can be picked up quickly. Researchers are also seeking alternative materials from which to make implants.

How long do silicone implants last?

Silicone implants do not wear out. If you have an implant it will only be necessary to change it if you put on or lose weight or develop a capsular contracture (formation of tough, fibrous tissue around the implant) which may cause problems. It is very difficult to damage implants – only a very severe chest injury would do this. So you can carry on with all your normal activities, including things like sports and air travel, without worrying about your implant.

Among the newer implants under evaluation are those using triglyceride oil, sometimes referred to as soya implants. These have the advantage of being processed by the body in the same way as vegetable oils, and may resist bacterial and fungal infection.

Breast reconstruction using muscle and skin flaps

This type of breast reconstruction uses flaps of muscle and skin which are generally taken from the back or abdomen. These areas of the body contain very large muscles, providing enough skin and muscle for reconstruction of a breast form on the chest wall. The large muscle used from the back is called the *latissimus dorsi* muscle and the muscle from the abdomen is the *rectus abdominis* muscle (see diagrams on pages 16 and 18).

This type of procedure is appropriate for women in whom tissue expansion has proved unsuccessful or is unsuitable because a lot of skin and muscle has been removed from the breast. It may also be useful where previous radiotherapy has made the skin unsuitable for tissue expansion.

Breast reconstruction using muscle and skin from the back

There will be a scar on the back and another oval one around the reconstructed breast.

Using the muscle (latissimus dorsi) and skin from the back

One technique for this type of operation involves rotating a flap of muscle and overlying skin from the back directly behind the operated breast, together with its own blood supply. The flap is tunnelled to just below the armpit and repositioned on the chest wall.

Usually there is not enough tissue to form the breast mound so an implant may be placed behind it to match the size of the other breast.

This type of operation leaves scars both from where the skin and muscle flap is taken and on the reconstructed breast. The scar around the reconstructed breast is oval and the scar on the back is usually horizontal, so it can generally be covered by a bra. Sometimes this scar is more diagonal which can make it more difficult to cover with a bra. Ask your surgeon what type of scar will result in your case.

Using the muscle (rectus abdominis) and skin from the abdomen

A flap of muscle with its overlying skin is taken from the large abdominal muscle. It is then rotated and tunnelled upwards from the abdomen and placed on the chest wall to create a breast form. There is usually enough tissue provided by this technique to match the remaining breast. Sometimes an implant is needed to achieve the right size.

This type of operation is sometimes referred to as a TRAM flap because the Transverse Rectus Abdominis Muscle is used.

Scarring with this type of surgery may vary, as the scar on the abdomen can be vertical or horizontal. The scar around the breast will be oval.

Breast reconstruction using muscle and skin flap rotation, from the back or abdomen, is a major operation requiring a hospital stay of at least one week. Using a flap from the back generally poses less risk of complications but will often require use of an implant.

Breast reconstruction using muscle and skin from the abdomen

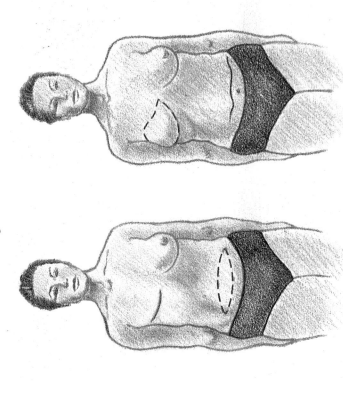

The scar on the abdomen will be from side to side, as shown here, or vertical. The scar on the breast will be oval.

Example of a breast reconstruction using an implant.
With nipple reconstruction

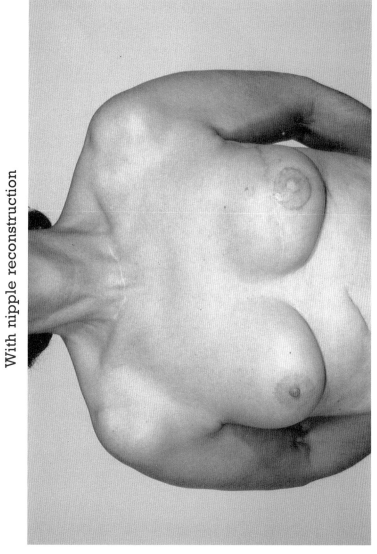

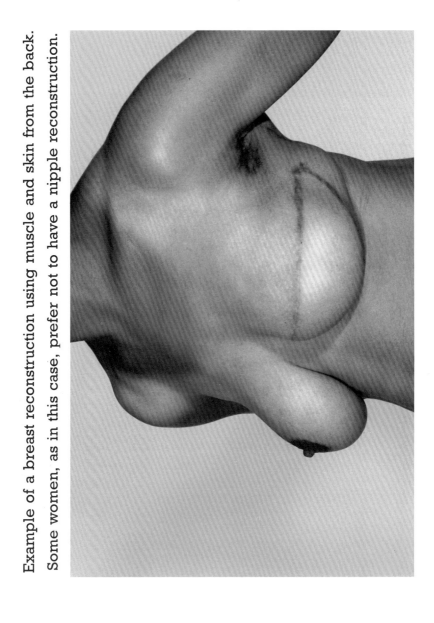

Example of a breast reconstruction using muscle and skin from the back. Some women, as in this case, prefer not to have a nipple reconstruction.

Example of a breast reconstruction using muscle and skin from the abdomen. With nipple reconstruction.

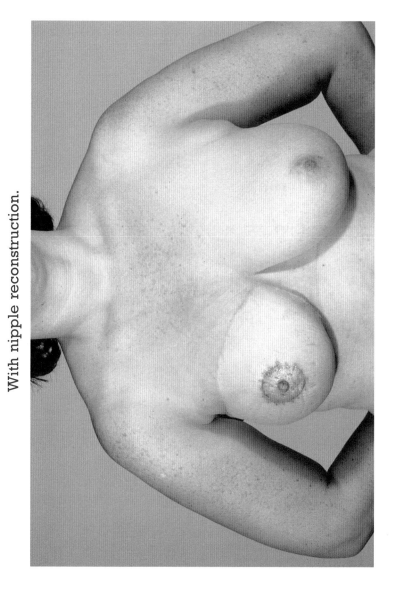

A positive result

After surgery for breast cancer this young woman underwent breast reconstruction. This photograph was taken at her wedding a few months later. Two years later, she is well and expecting their first baby.

A third type of tissue transfer method uses tissue from the buttocks. It is only considered suitable in a few cases.

Reconstructing the nipple

The reconstructed breast obviously does not have a nipple if this has been removed during mastectomy or lumpectomy. But it is possible to have a nipple reconstructed on the breast reconstruction. This is usually done some time after the breast reconstruction has healed and settled into its final shape and position. This enables the surgeon to position the nipple accurately, in line with the one on your other breast. The time interval between the two operations – for breast and nipple reconstruction – may vary, but is usually about three to four months.

Techniques used

Surgeons use various techniques for nipple reconstruction. The nipple may be reconstructed from grafted skin tissue, taken from other suitable areas of your body. Two areas which may be used are the nipple and areola from the remaining natural breast and the top of the inner thigh, where the skin is darker in colour. Alternatively, a 'tattooing' technique may be used on the peak of the new breast to produce a nipple. This however does not produce the shape beneath clothes.

It is important to be realistic about what to expect from a reconstructed nipple – it will not function or have the same sensation as a natural nipple.

Preserving the nipple

It may be possible to preserve the nipple if you are having immediate reconstruction. Your own nipple will be grafted onto the reconstructed breast. Alternatively, it may be possible to save the nipple by grafting it to another part of the body such as the abdomen or the upper thigh until surgery is carried out and then attach it to the reconstructed breast. The possibility of retaining your original nipple will depend on whether the surgeon thinks it, or attached tissue, may contain cancer cells.

You may decide that you do not want to undergo a second operation. In this case you could consider a silicone stick-on nipple which can be attached to the reconstructed breast. These can be purchased ready-made or made to match your other nipple, although this can be expensive.

Surgery to the other breast

Surgeons carrying out breast reconstruction aim to match the size and shape of the reconstructed breast to your remaining breast. But this is not always possible, so it may be suggested that an operation be performed on your natural breast to achieve a better match. This may involve reducing the size of your remaining breast or lifting it to reduce its natural droop. In some cases, it may be necessary to remove and reposition the nipple.

This type of surgery will cause some scarring, but this will fade to some degree with time. Repositioning the nipple may lead to reduction or loss of sensation.

What can you expect from breast reconstruction?

Every effort is made to achieve the best possible result from reconstruction. But results from this type of surgery vary a great deal. It is impossible to achieve a perfect match with your natural breast, but the result of reconstruction can be very acceptable, giving you an 'equal' appearance when wearing a bra.

When undressed you may find that the reconstructed breast has less of a droop and appears more proud and firmer to the touch than your natural breast. There is often much less sensation in the reconstructed breast.

The examples on the following pages give some idea of what can be achieved.

If the shape of the reconstructed breast differs greatly from your natural breast even when wearing underwear it is possible to insert a partial prosthesis into your bra to look more balanced. Breast prostheses come in a wide range of shapes, sizes and skin colours. They are made of soft silicone, which can reproduce the natural curves of your breast, including the nipple outline. A well-fitting prosthesis restores your balance as well as your shape.

The pictures of breast reconstructions on pages 19-21 do not necessarily show what is possible in your case. Many factors can influence the result. A member of the team caring for you, such as the breast care nurse, could put you in touch with other women who have had the operation, if you would like to talk to them.

Recovery after breast reconstruction

Immediately after surgery your reconstructed breast will be covered with dressings, which nursing staff will change regularly. At first, your new breast will be larger than your other breast, but it should reduce in size over a few weeks.

Once your doctor tells you it is healed, you can bathe or take showers. These will help to keep your wounds clean. Showers may be better than baths because soaking may increase the risk of infection in the wound, but avoid a direct spray of water onto your reconstructed breast. Wash with lukewarm water and nonperfumed soap, rinsing the wound line well. Pat the wound area dry with a clean towel – do not rub it.

Massaging the skin over the reconstruction

Surgeons generally advise women to massage the skin over the reconstruction daily with body oil or cream. This keeps the skin supple and in good condition. The massaging action will also reduce the risk of encapsulation (formation of a tough, fibrous coat) around an implant.

Wearing a bra after reconstructive surgery

Some surgeons advise women to wear a support garment, usually a firm, supportive bra, for several weeks after reconstructive surgery. They may recommend wearing this at night as well as during the day. Other surgeons consider this is unnecessary and suggest wearing a normal bra, or no bra at all. They believe that this encourages a more natural droop of the reconstructed breast and that wearing a bra makes little difference to the cosmetic results of surgery.

Arm movement after breast reconstruction

By about six weeks after breast reconstruction you should have regained full range of movement with little discomfort in the arm nearest the reconstructed breast. It is important that immediately after surgery a physiotherapist shows you how to carry out suitable arm exercises. The recommended exercises will be changed as you recover.

Some surgeons recommend specific exercise regimes after reconstructive surgery. Check with your surgeon what is right for you.

Psychological adjustment

The change in your breast shape will take some time for you to get used to. You will have already had a lot to cope with, with the initial diagnosis, treatment and surgery for breast cancer. This is yet another stage. At first your new breast might not really feel like 'you' – it will take some time to get used to your new shape.

Radiotherapy after breast reconstruction

It is possible to have radiotherapy following breast reconstruction, but it would not be carried out while a tissue expander was being inflated. This is because radiotherapy reduces the ability of your skin to stretch. It will also delay skin healing. So any necessary radiotherapy is given prior to inflation or, if medical advice permits, delayed until the implant has been fully inflated.

Possible complications after breast reconstruction

Many women who have had a breast removed because of cancer now undergo reconstructive surgery. As growing numbers of reconstructive operations have been carried out techniques and implants have improved. Nowadays the complications are much less than they used to be. However, there are still some risks connected with any type of surgery and a few connected particularly with breast reconstruction. It is best to be prepared for these possible problems to help you cope with them if they occur.

Problems associated with any type of surgery which may occur after breast reconstruction include: bleeding, problems associated with having a general anaesthetic, collection of fluid under the wound, pain and discomfort, and excessive scar tissue (keloid scarring).

Immediate problems

Wound infection

This is a rare complication of any type of surgery. If it occurs antibiotics can usually get rid of the infection. In a very few cases infection may persist despite antibiotics. If an implant has been used it may have to be removed in order to treat the infection successfully. In this situation, doctors generally advise waiting for a few months before having another implant inserted or undergoing a different type of reconstruction.

Inspect your wound (incision line) regularly once you are back at home after surgery. Tell your breast care nurse or doctor immediately if you have any of the following:

- increased redness or change in colour over the breast, around the scar area, or both
- discharge (fluid being released) from incisions
- a fever, with your temperature going above 38°C (100.5°F).

Collection of fluid under the wound

After breast reconstructive surgery you will have drainage tubes inserted into the wound to drain away any fluid that may collect. These are long, thin, plastic tubes attached to vacuum drainage bottles. They are usually removed several days after your operation. However, after the removal of the drains a collection of fluid (a seroma) or blood (a haematoma) sometimes develops under the wound. These may be absorbed by the body if they are small, but if they are large they may need to be removed by a surgeon using a small needle and syringe.

Pain and discomfort

After any type of operation you are likely to feel some pain and discomfort. Women vary greatly in how much pain they suffer after breast reconstruction. Some may need painkilling injections for a day or so after surgery. But most women report that the procedure is less painful than they expected and find they can control the discomfort by taking pain-killing tablets for a few days. Make sure you ask for pain-relieving drugs if you need them. There is no need to suffer in silence – in fact, research suggests that patients with good pain relief recover more quickly after surgery.

Itching is a sensation that often accompanies wound healing, so you may feel this where incisions have been made. This may be very uncomfortable, but it is obviously important not to scratch the healing skin. The itching will decrease as the wound heals. You may find it uncomfortable moving the arm on the side where surgery has been carried out. This is particularly likely if you have reconstruction at the same time as surgery for breast cancer and have had some lymph glands removed from your armpit. But it is important that you continue using your arm and carry out exercises suggested by your physiotherapist.

After immediate breast reconstruction (carried out at the same time as breast cancer surgery) you may feel **tingling sensations** down your arm on the side of the new breast. You may also have some **numbness** in the upper and inner arm. This is an effect of the surgery on the nerves in that area. It will gradually fade over time but may last up to a year after surgery.

If your reconstruction involved taking tissue from your abdomen, you will find bending and stretching uncomfortable for a few weeks after surgery. Supporting your wound with your hands when you bend should help.

Possible longer-term problems

Capsular contracture

When any foreign body such as an implant is put into your body, your immune system responds by forming fibrous tissue around it. Over a few months this fibrous tissue will contract as part of the natural healing process. If this contraction is severe then you may experience tightening, hardening and changes in the shape of the reconstructed breast, which may be uncomfortable and spoil the match with your natural breast. Up to one in three women having a breast implant may suffer this problem, although recent improvements in the technique have reduced the risk. Most capsular contractions form in the first year but some may take up to 3 years.

In a few cases the implant and capsule may have to be surgically removed. A replacement implant can then be inserted at the same time. The risk of developing a capsular contracture that requires further surgery is between one in five and one in ten.

Asymmetry (unequal appearance of the breasts)

Your surgeon will try to create a breast form that matches your own breast as closely as possible. But it is not possible to achieve a perfect match. Capsular contraction may improve the match, so you need to wait for some months after surgery to assess the final results. It may also be possible to improve the degree of match by putting on or losing weight. If you find the lack of symmetry unacceptable, discuss this with your breast care nurse or doctor. It may be possible to improve it by having surgery on your other breast or by replacing the implant with another that is a different size, or is positioned slightly differently.

Other complications

Abdominal hernia is a rare complication following a TRAM flap. This is due to removal of the abdominal muscle, which may weaken the abdominal wall. If this is a risk your surgeon may insert a protective mesh to replace the muscle and prevent this happening.

Using a flap from your back (latissimus dorsi) may reduce your shoulder movement, because of the loss of muscle. Sometimes, women may find they suffer muscle weakness in the affected shoulder and may have less strength in their arm.

Finding a surgeon

It is essential to find a reputable and highly experienced surgeon to carry out breast reconstruction. First of all, ask your breast cancer surgeon if there is anyone in their hospital who performs breast reconstruction. If there is not, he or she may be able to recommend another doctor in your region. It may be difficult to get a referral because a limited number of surgeons perform breast reconstruction operations.

Before you visit any surgeon you might like to ask your GP about the surgeon's qualifications, experience and reputation in breast reconstruction surgery. You need a surgeon who is experienced in the particular type of operation you will be having.

You should also feel confident that the surgeon is sensitive to the thoughts and feelings of someone who is having breast reconstruction.

Some questions to ask your surgeon

It may be useful to take this list of questions, in addition to others you think of, to help you gain the information you need to consider before deciding to have breast reconstruction.

- What type of surgery would you recommend for me? Why?
- What are the risks and benefits associated with this?
- What is your experience in this type of surgery?
- May I see photographs of other patients who have had breast reconstruction carried out by you?
- What can I expect my reconstructed breast to look and feel like? Immediately after surgery? After 6 months? After one year?
- How long will I need to stay in hospital?
- How long will it take me to recover?
- What do I need to do to ensure a good recovery?
- When can I have surgery?

(You can use the fill-in form facing the inside back cover of this booklet to note the questions you want to ask and the answers you receive).

Checking your breasts after reconstruction

It is vital to continue checking both your remaining natural breast and the area of your reconstructed breast after surgery. If you have not previously done this, ask your nurse to show you how to examine your breasts. There are information leaflets available which show you how to do it. Your doctor will also regularly examine your breasts after your reconstruction.

Things to look out for during breast self-examination include:

- tissue feels different – harder or tighter
- the appearance or shape changes
- a change in skin texture – puckering, dimpling, rash, thickening
- visible lump or bulge
- lump or lumpy area you can feel in either breast or armpit
- the nipple turns in or points differently
- discharge from the nipple of any kind
- rash or swelling on the nipple or the areola (the dark area around the nipple)
- enlarged glands under either armpit
- swelling of the upper arm
- pain or discomfort that feels different to tenderness before your periods.

Tell your nurse or doctor if you find anything which concerns you.

Mammography after reconstruction

Your doctor will advise you on whether mammography is still suitable for your reconstructed breast. If you have had all the breast tissue removed you will probably not need mammograms for the reconstructed breast – although you will still have them for the natural breast.

Silicone or saline implants hide part of the breast during mammography, but experts believe any cancer around an implant is still simple to detect. Your doctor can advise you on how any possible recurrence of cancer will be picked up.

Common questions

Q. What does a reconstructed breast look like?

A reconstructed breast will not look exactly the same as a natural breast, but differences should not be noticeable when wearing clothes. The new breast may look flatter or more youthful than your natural breast.

Q. Does a reconstructed breast feel different?

Breast implants are designed to feel like a natural breast, being soft and pliable. They are similar in weight and density to breast tissue, so you should feel a balance between the reconstructed breast and your remaining breast. The implant may move slightly, so the reconstructed breast may have some 'bounce'.

The skin over your reconstructed breast will feel normal to the touch because it's your own skin, but sensations in the surgical area will probably be less than normal.

Q. How good is the match with my natural breast?

Surgeons make every possible effort to match the remaining breast, but a reconstructed breast is unlikely to be an exact duplicate in size, shape or outline. The same is true for a reconstructed nipple.

If you are concerned about lack of matching your surgeon may suggest modifying your natural breast to give a more balanced appearance. The most common procedures carried out are reduction, enlargement or lifting of the natural breast.

Q. What if I am not happy with the results?

Your level of satisfaction with breast reconstruction will depend mainly on what you expect before the surgery. Make sure you discuss your expectations with your surgeon before you decide to proceed. It is important to wait for several months after reconstruction for the skin and muscle to stretch and for the reconstructed breast to settle into its final shape before deciding how happy you are with the result. If you then have concerns, discuss them with your surgeon or breast care nurse.

Q. Could a breast implant hide a new cancer?

Specialists consider there is little or no difficulty in detecting a recurrence of cancer either beneath or around an implant, using examination by hand or mammography (X-rays of the breast). If cancer returns, it is most likely to be just under the skin so should be easy to detect.

Q. Do implants cause cancer?

No. Latest medical research shows there is no evidence that they cause cancer.

Q. Does breast reconstruction interfere with other treatments (such as radiotherapy or chemotherapy)?

Immediate reconstruction will not make either of these treatments less effective. But treatment is often delayed to allow healing of the surgery.

Q. Is breast reconstruction available on the NHS?

Yes. If you have had or are going to have a mastectomy as cancer treatment, you are entitled to free breast reconstruction on the NHS. Alternatively, some surgeons will carry out reconstructive surgery privately, if you prefer.

BACUP's Cancer Support Service

Information

Provides information on all aspects of cancer and its treatment, and on the practical and emotional problems of living with the illness. Information is on computer about services available to cancer patients, treatment and research centres, support groups, therapists, counsellors, financial assistance, insurance, mortgages and home nursing services. Some of these are listed on the following pages.

If you would like any other help, you can phone and speak to one of our experienced cancer nurses. The service is open to telephone enquiries from 9am to 7pm Monday to Friday. The number to call is 0171 613 2121. You can call the information service free of charge on 0800 18 11 99.

Counselling

Many people feel that counselling can help them deal with the problems of living with cancer. Counsellors use their skills to help people talk through the emotional difficulties linked to cancer. These are not always easy to talk about and are often hardest to share with those to whom you are closest. Talking with a trained counsellor who is not personally involved can help to untangle thoughts, feelings and ideas.

BACUP's cancer counselling service can give information about local counselling services and can discuss with people whether counselling could be appropriate and helpful for them. BACUP runs a one-to-one counselling service based at its London and Glasgow offices.

For more information about counselling, or to make an appointment please ring 0171 696 9000 (London), or 0141 553 1553 (Glasgow).

Booklets

For a list of BACUP booklets, or to order another BACUP booklet, phone 0171 696 9003.

Useful organisations

BACUP
3 Bath Place
Rivington Street
London
EC2A 3JR
Office: 0171 696 9003

BACUP Scotland
Cancer Counselling Service
30 Bell Street
Glasgow
G1 1LG
Office: 0141 553 1553

Information
0171 613 2121 or Freephone 0800 18 11 99
Open 9am-7pm Monday-Friday

Counselling
London: 0171 696 9000
Glasgow: 0141 553 1553

All BACUP's London numbers can take minicom calls.

Jersey BACUP
6 Royal Crescent, St Helier, Jersey JE2 4QG
Tel: 01534 490085 Freephone: 0800 735 0275

*In addition to providing a link with BACUP's Cancer
Information Service in the Channel Islands, Jersey BACUP runs
a local cancer support group and trained local volunteers
give support over the telephone, and in the local hospital.*

Breast Cancer Care
Kiln House, 210 New King's Road, London SW6 4NZ
Tel: 0171 384 2984
Suite 2/8, 65 Bath Street, Glasgow G2 2BX
Tel: 0141 353 1050
Free national helpline: 0500 245 345

*Gives information, emotional support and practical advice to
women who have or fear they have breast cancer. Has a
national volunteer support service, a helpline, and a
prosthesis-fitting service, with a selection of bras and
swimwear in the London and Glasgow offices.*

Cancer Care Society
21 Zetland Road, Redland, Bristol BS6 7AH
Tel: 0117 942 7419

Provides counselling and emotional support where possible through a network of support groups around the country. Holiday accommodation is available, and in some areas hospital visiting and help with transport.

CancerLink
11-21 Northdown Street, London N1 9BN
Tel: 0800 132 905 (Freephone helpline)

Offers support and information on all aspects of cancer in response to telephone and letter enquiries. Acts as a resource to cancer support and self-help groups throughout the UK, and publishes a range of publications on issues about cancer.

Macmillan Cancer Relief
Anchor House, 15-19 Britten Street, London SW3 3TZ
Tel: 0171 351 7811
(With regional offices throughout the country)

Provides specialist advice and support through Macmillan nurses and doctors and financial grants for people with cancer and their families.

Marie Curie Cancer Care
28 Belgrave Square, London SW1X 8QG
Tel: 0171 235 3325

Runs eleven hospice centres for cancer patients throughout the UK, and a community nursing service which works in conjunction with the district nursing service to support cancer patients and their carers in their homes.

Tak Tent Cancer Support – Scotland
Block C20, Western Court, 100 University Place,
Glasgow G12 6SQ
Tel: 0141 211 1932

Offers information, support, education and care for cancer patients, families, friends and professionals. Network of support groups throughout Scotland. 'Drop-in' resource and information centre at the above address.

Tenovus Cancer Information Centre
PO Box 88, College Buildings, Courtenay Road, Splott,
Cardiff CF1 1SA
Tel: 01222 497700
     0800 526527 (Freephone helpline)

Provides an information service in English and Welsh on all aspects of cancer, and emotional support for cancer patients and their families. Operates a mobile screening unit, drop-in centre, support group and cancer helpline.

The Ulster Cancer Foundation
40-42 Eglantine Avenue, Belfast BT9 6DX
Tel: 01232 663439 (helpline)
     01232 663281 (admin)

Provides a cancer information helpline and resource centre, and support groups for patients and relatives.

Recommended reading

Michael Baum, Christobel Saunders and Sheena Meredith
Breast cancer: a guide for every woman
Oxford University Press, 1994   ISBN 0 19 262436 9   £8.99
Includes a section about breast reconstruction: descriptions
of the different techniques, with photographs.

Robert Buckman
*What you really need to know about cancer: a comprehensive
guide for patients and their families*
Macmillan, 1996   ISBN 0 333 61866 1   £20.00
Chapters on all types of cancer including breast cancer.
Sections on conventional and complementary treatments,
screening, living with cancer and attitudes to cancer.

Carolyn Faulder
Breast cancer and breast care
Ward Lock (in association with Breast Cancer Care), 1995
ISBN 0 7063 7411 8   £6.99
Information on breast cancer treatments and rehabilitation,
including breast reconstruction. The different techniques of
breast reconstruction are described and illustrated.

The Royal Marsden Hospital
Breast reconstruction (Patient Information Series: No. 23)
Royal Marsden, 1990   ISBN 0 949015 22 9   £1.50
A brief overview of common methods of breast
reconstruction.

Diana Moran
A more difficult exercise
Bloomsbury, 1989   ISBN 0 7475 0349 4   £12.95
Diary of the 'green goddess', who has had a double
mastectomy and reconstructive surgery.

Val Speechley and Maxine Rosenfield
*Cancer information at your fingertips: the comprehensive
cancer reference book for the 1990s* (2nd edn)
Class Publishing, 1996   ISBN 1 872362 56 7   £11.95
Questions and answers about cancer, its diagnosis,
treatment, side effects, complementary therapies and life
with cancer.

Questions you might like to ask your doctor or surgeon

You can fill this in before you see the doctor or surgeon, and then use it to remind yourself of the questions you want to ask, and the answers you receive.

1. ....

Answer ....

....

2. ....

Answer ....

....

3. ....

Answer ....

....

4. ....

Answer ....

....

5. ....

Answer ....

....

6. ....

Answer ....

....